100 Easy but Powerful Diet Habits

Powerful, Healthy Habits that lead to major weight loss and change your life

Anna G Taylor

Table of Contents

INTRODUCTION

Thank you, and congratulations on picking up "100 Easy Habits for Weight Loss" on your Ereader. The following tips and tricks, as they were, are designed to help aid you in losing weight and becoming generally healthier over time and to generally feel better throughout your day, week, and life.

The following 100 habits range from eating and exercise, to the proper times to perform a number of acts throughout the day, to simple adjustments you can make to your daily routine to make the most out of anything you do. These are designed to keep you healthy physically, mentally, and emotionally to keep you at the peak of your game and feeling great!

It should be noted that you can't expect results after one day of participating in any or all of the habits listed in this book. They are "habits," after all, meaning you will need to put in some effort to make these activities part of your everyday life.

As an additional bonus, some "habits" are placed under some sample healthy recipes for you to try at the end of the book. A major habit that will help you lose weight over time (and arguably the easiest and most natural habit that everyone should make) is cooking proper food. The recipes included in this book are relatively easy to make and are here for you to try your hand at cooking healthier meals.

As a bonus to that bonus, learning to use your time you spend cooking or preparing food is also an easy way to remain healthy mentally. You may wonder how that makes sense at this point in your reading. Read on to learn several habits that can be used doing usually mundane tasks (like cooking or preparing food).

Once these habits do become a part of your routine, you'll start to notice changes to your health. So, enjoy and good luck!

Chapter 1: A Healthy Mindset

The first part to forming any habit (bad or good) is how you approach it. These first several tips are here for you to apply to all other habits you form throughout your life to make the most of their potential (or to limit any bad effects the bad habits may come with).

Habit #1: Stay Mindful of Your Actions

Too easily can we fall into a routine with too many bad routines in it. This can range anything from eating out too many times a week because you don't want to spend the time to cook to buying things on impulse because "hey, I've got a few extra dollars, so what's the harm?" While spontaneity is not intrinsically a bad thing, making decisions without considering them first can lead to a lack of understanding of the consequences.

When making a decision, one that may lead to a habit down the road, stay in the present and consider it. If you don't think about something as you're doing it (like buying fast food for dinner four times a week) it will become a habit without you even realizing it.

It works for good habits, too. Yes, waking up early on a Sunday morning to run in the cold is difficult, but if you stay in the present and remind yourself why you want to run, you'll find it easier to drag yourself out of bed. If you don't stay aware of the present, you'll find yourself pulling the covers over your head and falling right back to sleep.

Here's the kicker: Staying present and mindful of the situation or decision at hand is also a habit you have to force yourself to learn. So stay mindful of staying mindful and the rest just may fall into place.

Habit #2: Mindfulness of Your Thoughts

Mindfulness doesn't only affect how you view your actions, it also impacts how you think about your own thinking.

It's important to reflect on your thoughts throughout the day to understand your mind better and to change any harmful habits you may have. If you find yourself having negative thoughts about your habits, staying mindful of these thoughts will help you identify them and change them before it harms your progress toward a healthier you.

Your own thoughts about your habits or progress toward a healthier you are self-fulfilling prophesies. That is, whatever you believe about yourself will eventually happen. It's important to stay positive about your progress and understand that you may not see results right away, but if you keep telling yourself that you are getting healthier, the results will come after.

If, on the other hand, you keep telling yourself that you won't get any healthier because you can't see the results right away, you'll be more likely to give up and then definitely won't see any results.

Once you've moved past your doubts, you can begin to visualize your desired outcome. If you want to lose ten pounds, constantly visualize yourself losing ten pounds to help you continue your routine. If you visualize yourself staying how you are, you won't make progress.

Your mind is a powerful tool, don't let it work against you to prevent you from achieving your goals. Use it to your advantage.

Habit #3: Know The Reason You're Doing Something

It's easy to break a habit if you don't have a personal reason to keep doing it. It's imperative that you make of a habit of doing things with a purpose in mind to keep you motivated and enthusiastic.

To keep your spirits high, consider what got you interested in the activity in the first place. If you want to run in the morning, understand what that means for you: you'll be in better shape, you'll wake up earlier, and you'll have more energy throughout the day. Those are specifically biological side effects of running everyday and work to inspire you to keep doing it. Your specific reason doesn't have to be so based in science, though. Maybe you want to eat healthier because a friend needs to eat better for their health, or maybe you just want to be able to fit into the tuxedo or dress of your dreams for your wedding. Whatever your reason, keep it in mind as you work on your habit to keep you working toward your goal.

Here's a fun tip that a lot of people tend to shy away from: Your reason is yours alone, so make it as selfish as you want. You don't need an altruistic reason to start being healthier, so find your reason for becoming healthier and stick to it. (It's also not a sin to want to be healthier for the sake of being healthier; It's as good a reason as any.)

Habit #4: Don't Make Excuses

On the flip side to having a reason for sticking to a habit, bad habits often have an excuse attached to keep you doing it. You may tell yourself "picking up fast food on the way home from work or school is easier and I'm too tired to cook." That's a fair point, it is easier to pick up fast food when you're driving home, but that doesn't make it a good reason.

Often times bad habits form from a lack of a good habit. If you make it a habit to come home from work or school everyday and make a meal for yourself, it will seem less and less like a chore and more and more like a fun part of your daily routine.

The tricky part of the reason-excuse dynamic is that sometimes it can be difficult to decide if your habit is backed by a good reason or a silly excuse. That's why it's important to always stay mindful of your decisions. Really consider your habits and think about why you're doing it rather than something else. You can easily rationalize fast food's ease and lack of time commitment, but that doesn't make it a good reason. In this case, the health detriments outweigh the benefits of saving half an hour to make dinner.

Habit #5: Make a Schedule and Stick to it

What makes a habit a habit is the fact that you do it constantly without thinking having to force yourself into starting it. The only way to do this is to create a daily (or weekly) schedule and to force yourself to stick to it. The more you stick to your schedule, the easier it will be for you to stick to your schedule.

With technology today, creating and sticking to a schedule has never been easier. Smartphones are perfect for creating a calendar with alarms to go off up to a day before your activity is planned, so you can have plenty of time to pump yourself up.

Some of the best advice I've ever been given is also the simplest in theory: Set an alarm for when you need to do something.

When the alarm goes off, do the task without hesitation.

If you have an alarm set for your daily tasks (waking up, going to work, cleaning the kitchen, mowing the lawn, homework, the list is limitless) and do that task as soon as the alarm goes off, you'll have a much easier time creating habits and keeping them. Like all things, it's easy to make an excuse for not doing it at the time, but if you force yourself to get up and do whatever your alarm says to do, you won't have time to consider all of the countless excuses not to do it.

Habit #6: Decide on Which Habits to Keep and Keep Them

Once you've thought long and hard about your habit and decided it was worth continuing, you then need to do just that: continue with it. There will be days where you want to skip a habit (no running on rainy days is probably a decent excuse), but that shouldn't mean you get to sleep in.

What most people don't consider is, oftentimes healthy habits tend to overlap. If one of your habits is running in the morning, then chances are another habit is waking up early. If, one day, you decide to not run for whatever reason and sleep in, you're breaking two of your habits with one fell swoop. While this isn't the worst thing to do every once in a while, doing this continually will lead to both of these habits falling out at the same time.

If you must skip one habit every now and again, make sure to keep up with your other habits to prevent yourself from not doing multiple healthy habits. If you do decide that today is not the day to wake up early and run, wake up at your normal time and consciously decide on another activity to fill that space (read, clean, spend extra time to cook a nice breakfast, etc.).

Habit #7: Stick to Your Habits

This may go without saying for many of you readers, but habits aren't formed after only one or two days. For the first while, you're going to have to force yourself to do whatever you want to make into a habit. On most of those days, you probably will hate it, but it gets easier after that first struggle.

On average, it takes about 21 days for an individual task to become a habit. That's three weeks of doing something that, honestly, you probably won't enjoy too much to reach a point where you can stand it. It's hard and can suck, but if you remind yourself of your reasons for doing it and stick to the schedule, you'll get to the point where you can't live without your habit.

Once you form a habit over those three weeks of pushing yourself, you may not fully appreciate how easy the task becomes. You may still hate running in the morning because of how hard it can be to wake up early. But, I promise you, once you get a habit locked in place, you won't be able to go a day or two without it without feeling the negative effects of not doing it.

It comes down to one thing to form a habit: Tenacity. It's all about pushing yourself to continue a task even when it's difficult to make it a habit in your everyday life. The aforementioned tips and tricks are designed specifically to make being tenacious easier and, therefore, making forming and keeping habits easier.

Chapter 2: Exercise Habits

Of course one of the best ways to stay in shape is to exercise. Most people attempt to fit in a few hours at the gym a few times a week to make sure they're getting the most for their time (and the most for their money seeing as most gyms come with a pretty hefty fee). Obviously, this is a decent method to lose some weight and put on some muscle, but that's a big time commitment and simply isn't for everyone.

Another option is to simply follow a few daily habits to keep you healthier in general. Sure, you may not get to the point where you will be able to bench press several hundred pounds, but with these habits you'll look and feel a lot healthier.

Habit #8: Wake Up Early

I know, I know, many of you readers out there don't consider yourself "morning people." I hate to tell you this, but the concept of someone being a natural morning person is a myth.

All your friends and coworkers you hate before 10 am because of how chipper they are aren't naturally that happy in the morning. They've allowed their body to adjust to waking up earlier which makes it easier for them to get up earlier.

The biggest key to changing your sleep schedule is not when you go to bed. You can go to bed at 7 pm to try to wake up earlier, but if your body is used to waking up at 9, it's going to try to wake up at 9. The most important variable is when you force yourself to wake up. If you set your alarm for 5:30 in the morning, force yourself to get out of bed at 5:30 and you'll find that in no time, you'll wake up around that time naturally.

Habit #9: Do Not Rely on Coffee or Caffeine

Too many people rely on caffeine to wake up in the morning. You know the types: "I haven't had my coffee yet, so I might yell at you." While some of them may be exaggerating a bit, a lot of people have trained their body to not properly function without their daily dose (or five) of coffee.

While coffee and energy drinks are inherently a negative, if you drink something with caffeine in it to start every single morning, your body loses its ability to create the proper chemicals to wake you up. Drinking coffee means the drink is doing the work for your body so it doesn't need to do it any longer. That means, it won't even try to wake you up if the coffee will do it instead.

All honestly, this isn't exactly an exercise habit, as I'm sure you've all figured out. But, it lends itself to exercise habits because, while coffee is a good way to wake up in the morning…

Habit 10: Exercise Makes a Great Wake Up Call

Working out is not the way most people want to start their day. It's a lot of effort early in the morning and that's understandably not appealing. But the fact is, you don't need to run a marathon in the morning to get the benefits of its wake-up powers.

Habit #11: Small Workouts Will Go a Long Way

Start your day with a dozen or so push ups or sit ups, or a jog around the block. Each of these should take you less than ten minutes and will force your tired and achy body to kick into gear right away.

Just by exerting some effort in the wee hours of the morning (something as small as walking to your car, even), will get your body going and make the rest of your morning easier than you could ever imagine.

Habit #12: Don't Limit Exercise to a Specific Time of the Day

While, yes, I did say it was good to have a strict schedule (and it is very important to forming and keeping habits), if you find yourself with a few minutes here or there, use the time to exercise.

Like the last few habits, I don't mean running a marathon or lifting weights in your office. If you find yourself with ten minutes left in your lunch hour, why not take a walk around the building? It might not be the most exciting activity, but just moving your body will help get rid of that post-lunch need for a nap as well as give you a chance to enjoy some fresh air.

Habit #13: Be Conscious of Your Exercise

Before you ask: no, I don't mean count every calorie you burn. What a lot of people is simply count their steps throughout the day. Fitbits, Smartwatches, and a ton of phone apps count your steps throughout the day.

Keeping track of your steps is a great way to get an overview of how much you're doing throughout the day. Most apps or products give you a nice little graph to show your progress over time so you can adjust accordingly.

Habit #14: Set Goals

Like everything in life, setting goals is an easy and often times fun way to monitor your progress. Setting goals gives you a tangible number to work with so your goals don't have to be vague or confusing.

Goals can range anywhere from how many calories you want to burn, to how many steps you want to take in a day. It's as simple as that. There is not a need to reach a specific weight before a specific date, just tell yourself "I want to walk 2 miles everyday." There's no stress about meeting a deadline, and no real punishment. The worst that may happen is you'll need to walk a mile or so when you get home in the evening (which is not a bad way to spend twenty minutes or so every evening).

Habit #15: Have a Partner or a Group

Sure, setting goals for yourself to meet is fun and can keep you motivated, but five people all trying to meet the same goal can be even more so.

The more people you exercise with, the more flexible you can make your goals. You can make exercise competitive or cooperative to push the members in your group to exercise more and more.

The more people participating, the more motivating it will be for each member to do their best.

Habit #16: Walk

That's it. Walk. You need to go to the store for a can of soup you forgot to pick up? Walk the mile to grab it. Sure, it may take longer, but you'll be getting in some nice exercise while enjoying some time outside.

Habit #17: Park Farther Away

If you need to run errands or go to the store to pick up a few things, park a block away or at the back of the parking lot. Sure, it may not be a lot of extra exercise, but that extra two hundred steps can add up if you park farther away for many different errands.

Habit #18: Move More

Throughout the day, we do countless small tasks that are oftentimes boring and require very little thought. During these activities, make it a point to move your body more. Dance while you sweep the kitchen or jog instead of walking somewhere. You don't need to take longer with the task if you swing your hips in time with a song while you clean.

Habit #19: Find Natural Breaks in Activities

You can work out so easily while watching TV or playing video games without missing a single beat. During commercial breaks, or loading screens for video games, fit in a few push ups, sit ups, or jumping jacks. Your show or game won't be interrupted and you'll be getting in a nice little workout here and there.

This also helps if you put in extra thought to what channel you want to watch or what video game you want to play. Some have longer commercial breaks or loading screens meaning you can get in slightly longer workouts each time, which does add up.

Habit #20: Get Rid of Daily Naps

Naps feel great, but if they'll longer than about half an hour, they can really mess up your sleep schedule for that night. Instead of crawling into bed right after work, try doing a light exercise to get your blood flowing again.

You won't want to work out when you feel tired in the afternoon, but if you pull the strength to walk around the block, you'll feel wide awake and ready to take on the rest of the day.

Habit #21: Monitor Your Sleep Habits

Again, this one isn't directly an exercise habit, but it does tie-in. If you work out more, you'll notice better sleep at night with fewer interruptions throughout the night. It also works the opposite way, if you notice that you may not have gotten great sleep over the last few nights, you have a chance to analyze your days and find a reason.

Habit #22: Start Small

Easy way to form a habit is to ease yourself into it. If you start out trying to run a marathon, you'll probably find it a bit difficult, may hurt yourself, and not see any benefits. Starting off your exercise habit with something small like a 10-minute walk will let you build up to the more intense activities.

Habit #23: Plan Ahead

This one ties into making a schedule and sticking to it, but expands upon it a bit more. Plan your week ahead of time with time set aside for your potential exercise habits. Planning several days ahead will make your schedule easier to follow.

Even planning a single day at a time is better than no plan. If you wake up and plan your day, you'll at the very least have a schedule set for the following 24 hours. A week is generally better because it does allow you to plan several days at a time without over planning (because planning a month is a bit much).

Habit #24: Know How to Deal with Ups and Downs

No matter how positive and motivated you are, there will be times when you don't want to work on being healthier. Motivation wears out, it's inevitable. That's why it's essential you make a habit of dealing with the highs and lows of your habit forming.

You can counted the lows with several strategies. Having a group of peers, friends, or coworkers will help keep you motivated when your own motivation won't cut it.

Habit #25: Cope with the Lows of Habit Forming

In a weird meta-habit kind of way, it takes habits to form habits. It's important to make a habit of dealing with your less-than-motivational times.

As mentioned in Habit #31, having a group of peers to help guide you, will keep you motivated and pushing through the tough times. Honestly, a lot of the previously mentioned habits can help pull you through the tough times with flying colors.

Asking for help will inspire you, forming a group (contest or competitive) will give you a responsibility to someone other than yourself, etc. The most important habit is to get up and exercise as soon as your schedule dictates it. Without that sense of self-motivation, the other habits will not be as easy to form.

Habit #26: Learn to Ride the Highs

There will be days that you are more motivated than you've ever been. Those days, as you'll find, are usually few and far between but godsends all the same. When those days do come around, it's never a bad thing to ride that high and extend your workout.

Habit #27: Don't Try to Compensate

Hypothetically, say you miss a day or two of workout. Don't worry too much about it, it's not the worst thing to happen. Just pick up your routine the following day and keep it going.

Do not try to compensate for lost time. While a little extra exercise throughout the day is not a bad thing (in fact, it's a great thing), working out to make up for a missed workout is not a good way to think about it. If you feel guilty and want to extend your exercise time the next day, that's great! But the mindset is not the most healthy one.

Feeling guilty won't help you motivate yourself. Just accept you missed a day and don't fret it after that. Going along with that, pushing yourself harder the next day just to make it up also isn't healthy. It creates this sense of punishment, which is not the point of making habits.

The other option is, it creates a sense of "if I can't do it today, I'll do it twice tomorrow and it'll even out." This mindset can lead to a lax perspective on forming habits, which can lead to an easy excuse to miss days.

Habit #28: Mind Your Breathing

This is one of the easiest habits to do throughout the day, but it's also one of the easiest to not do if you don't think about it. Proper breathing is an important part of staying healthy and getting the most out of your workouts. There are two major steps to note your breathing.

Monitor how you breathe throughout the day and throughout your workout. You'll notice the obvious change in speed depending on what activity you may be doing at a given time. Monitoring on its own is not incredibly helpful, but it's a necessary step toward something much bigger.

Controlling your breathing comes next. Taking ten minutes a day to work on breathing exercises will help you fill your lungs more than most people usually do, which means more blood flow and a more awake you. Deep breathing expands your chest, calms your mind, and allows you to take a break from the stress that comes with the day.

As you exercise, and once you get used to keeping track of your breathing, you can slow your breaths after a particularly heavy workout to keep your heart rate down and keep you feeling better. Monitoring and controlling your breathing is a fine habit to have by itself, but helps all other exercise habits formed be the most efficient they can be.

Habit #29: Make a Habit of Warming Up

It happens all too often that people don't warm up because "it just takes up more time." While it's true that a warm up can add ten minutes to your exercise routine, it'll save you time (and aches and pains) down the road.

Warming up before a workout helps jumpstart your metabolism so that the main part of your exercise will be as efficient as it can be. Not only does it help your exercise be as beneficial as possible, it also helps prevent aches in your muscles as you do workout.

The myth that warm ups have to take a lot of time is also a pretty harmful myth. While, yes, warm ups can take a chunk of time to do well, if your exercise only entails running around the block, five minutes of stretching will be plenty to keep you safe while exercising. Warm ups help burn more calories and keep you safer when working out means that there's no reason not to do it.

Habit #30: Learn to Cool Down Efficiently

Like a good warm up, a nice, relaxing cool down will make the most of your workout. Cool downs are meant to slowly slow your heart rate. It can be damaging to go from a quickened heart beat to a resting heart beat too quickly. Cool downs offer your body a few minutes to gently slow your heart rate at a nice pace.

Cool downs also offer a chance to prevent any aches and pains the following day. If you've ever tried to run and then woke up the next day with sore calves, it's most likely because you didn't cool down properly.

Make a habit of warming up and cooling down to make keeping your exercise habits easier to start day after day.

Habit #31: Balance Your Exercise with Your Food Intake

If your goal when working out is to lose weight, it's imperative that you know how much you need to work out (how many calories you need to burn) to lose that weight. Of course, half of this habit is decided what foods you eat (your calorie intake), but we'll talk about that a bit later.

In short, the more weight you want to lose, the more calories you need to burn. This can be done in two basic ways: working out more often (more time) or participating in more active activities (more intensity). For best results, it's best to make a habit out of mixing high intensity exercises with longer, less intense exercises.

Forming this habit also means that you need to know your limits and you need to understand that results may not be apparent right away. If you don't fully grasp these two aspects to exercising, you run the risk of pushing yourself too hard and really injuring yourself.

Habit #32: Spend Money on Exercise-Based Games

It's always helpful to have fun while working out. There are dozens of games and apps that help guide you through workouts while keeping the exercises fun. If you have the proper hardware already, the prices will obviously be cheaper, but if you don't this may not be the best option.

Nintendo's Wii Fit has been used by thousands of people to work out and stay active in their own home. It offers a lot of essential aspects to make your experience exercising fun and personal. Different Games, workout history, Wii Fit Community, and a wide variety of workouts, stretches, and activities all keep your exercise time entertaining.

If you don't own a Nintendo Wii, there are apps on both android and iPhone that help make normal, everyday workouts a bit more. Some offer you rewards based on your exercise habits (like a level up system in a video game), other offer narratives to help push you to work out more.

The key to all workouts is to be willing to be flexible and trying different strategies until you find the system that works for you.

Habit #33: Pavlov your Exercises with Mouth-Watering Treats

Training yourself to exercise can take place on two levels: Conscious and Subconscious. If you're unfamiliar with Pavlov's dogs, the short story is a man would ring a bell whenever he fed his dogs. Then, when he would ring the bell without feeding his dogs, the animals' mouths would begin to water. Their brains were reprogrammed to think they were hungry whenever a bell rang.

You can do something similar to your brain. If you give yourself a reason to want to exercise, you can trick your mind into associating your work out with whatever treat you decide on.

A lot of people do this with what is known as a "runner's high." Once your body gets used to running (or exercising in general), your mind will create more dopamine which makes you feel happier and more energetic. It's very possible to associate exercising with this "runner's high," and like most highs, it's sought after and chased.

In short, you can convince your mind to start exercising to feel good during or after, making it much easier to start an exercise everyday.

Habit #34: Don't Allow Yourself to Get Too Far Off Track

If you do happen to miss a morning's worth of workouts, don't make the excuse that you'll get back to it tomorrow. If you have time later in the day, there's no harm in shifting your workout from the morning to the evening (don't make a habit of mixing your schedule around, though).

And, of course, there's always the common excuse of "I'll get back into my schedule after the holidays." Don't fall into this loop. The longer you stay away from your routine, the harder it will be to get back into it.

Habit #35: Tell Yourself What You're Going to Do

If you want to start working out in the morning, tell yourself the night before that you need to get up early to go for a run. If you remind yourself about your desired routine, you'll be more likely to do it. If you make a weekly plan which includes working out, reminding yourself of your routine will be much easier to do.

If you remind yourself throughout the day about your new routine and habits, you also don't run the risk of making plans that may disrupt your routine (which can lead to you falling out of your routine and breaking your new habits).

Habit #36: Let Momentum Build

If you're able to remind yourself of your new habits and routines, and not fall off track too much, you'll notice that your exercises become easier and easier as time goes on. The more consistent you are with your work out, the easier it will be to reach that "high" we talked about earlier, and the less likely you are to get off track. Momentum helps build habits and keep them.

Habit #37: Make Exercise Accessible

Simply put, the harder it is for you to start a workout, the more excuses you can make and the less likely you are to start. If you want to run in the morning, use basketball shorts as pajamas and place your running shoes by your bed. That way, you're ready to go as soon as you leave your room and will have no excuses not to run.

Alternatively, if you wash your shorts the night before but still need to dry them in the morning, that 30 minutes may be enough time for you to rationalize not going on a run. The easier it is for you to work out, the easier it will be for you to start working out.

Habit #38: Start as Soon as Possible

It's pretty cliche, but don't hold off until tomorrow, or Monday to start working out. Get up now and go on a walk or a run. Do fifteen pushups before moving on to the next habit. That's all there is to it.

The sooner you can make a new routine, the sooner you'll form new habits, and the sooner it will be easier to stick to those habits.

Habit #39: Starting is the Hardest Part

Get in the habit of starting your exercise no matter how much you don't want to. Once you start walking or lifting weights, you'll enjoy it more than you thought you would.

This ties in with several other habits present throughout this book. Starting is hardest if you haven't already formed the habit. If you participate in a habit day after day, each time it will get easier for you so, as I mention later in the book, keep your momentum going.

Habit #40: Use Inspirational Music

Nothing gets you pumped up quite like a fast-paced playlist on your phone or MP3 player. Use energetic songs to lift your spirits and motivate you.

Music can do a lot to change a person's mood. Classical music like Chopin can calm a person and slow their heart rate. While this is also a good habit (meditating and slowing down, that is), fast paced music also raises your heart rate and increases your willingness to get up and work out. Find or make a playlist utilizing hard rock, electronic, or even pop music to get you going.

Habit #41: Post Reminders

Don't rely on your phone's alarm, and definitely don't rely on your memory to remind yourself to exercise. Post notes or reminders in commonly used areas of your home to give you that extra bit of push toward the door.

This may seem a silly little thing, but it can make or break a habit. And, sure, you may need to explain to countless friends and family members why you have little yellow post-it notes on your walls, doors, and refrigerator, but seeing the little beacons all over your house (or at least on commonly used appliances or commonly seen surfaces) will keep you constantly reminded of the habits you're trying to form.

Habit #42: Always Take the Stairs

Unless you have a legitimate reason not to, there's no reason you shouldn't take the stairs. Often times, they'll get you to the right floor faster than the elevator can arrive and you'll get some well-earned burning calves as a reward.

Habit #43: Explore Your Surroundings on Foot

Even if you've lived in the same town all your life, there's no harm in taking to the sidewalks and exploring the city. You'll notice a different side to life when you step away from your car and take the time to walk around.

Habit #44: Don't Think of Exercise as a Chore

Your time to exercise is just that: your time. Consider it a break or time to reflect on your day. The worst part about exercise is that it can be so tiring and, many people believe, wear you out. While this is an understandable assumption, working out actually keeps you awake and energized throughout the day.

Habit #45: Drink Water

Drinking water itself isn't exercise itself, but it will help you stay in better shape, help you continue to exercise, and keep you overall healthier in the process.

Habit #46: Reflect on Your Workouts

Once you've finished your workout, look back and figure out what you enjoyed about it, and what you didn't like so much. What made you feel better after doing, and what tired you out too much?

Habit #47: Make Your Routine a Part of Your Life

Habits are habits once they become ingrained in your schedule. Exercise ritualistically until it become a basic part of your day to day life. This applies to all habits you're attempting to form. Eating healthy is another big one that can be easily broken like exercise. Just keep at it, deter temptation in whatever forms they may come, and keep at it.

Habit #48: Mark Your Progress

Exercise does bring some relatively instant benefits. Feeling healthier, having more energy, and working out easier are only a few benefits that can come right away from exercise. Note these small positives to keep you going until the larger benefits start to appear.

Many apps (including Fitbit and many others) show you a graph of progress. These apps can show you how many calories you burn, how many steps you take, or even your elevation throughout the day (equivalent to how many flights of stairs you walked up and down throughout the day). The best part about these apps is, if something keeps track of your progress, you won't have to.

Habit #49: Look for Events Around Town

There are always runs happening around the country for a multitude of reasons. From yearly Turkey Trots, to Color or Mud runs for charity, there are dozens of themes and reasons that a city or company may hold a run, so keep your eyes peeled.

All types of events can get you out and about. Film festivals downtown, fairs, pub crawls (to some degree), and other type events will help you stay off that couch and out in the real world. The more frequently you keep up with local events and happenings, the more events you'll discover and the more fun you'll have.

Habit #50: Find Others With Similar Goals

If you don't have any friends or acquaintances that want to exercise with you, find others in the surrounding area that will. Having similar exercise goals or hobbies is a great way to meet new people and expand your social circle.

It's always easier to work toward something with another person. Not only will you have someone to struggle with, and enjoy your new routines with, but you'll have another person to hold you accountable. With a friend, it no longer is only you with the responsibility to yourself. Now someone is responsible to you, and you're responsible to them.

Habit #51: Your House is a Natural Gym

Just because you don't own any pricey equipment, doesn't mean you can't work out at your house. Exercises like jumping jacks, push ups, sit ups, and even lifting chairs can make for a quick and easy way to get in a workout.

This works with other activities, too. If you have a staircase, walk up and down it twice instead of just going upstairs. If you have a lawn, keeping it well-trimmed and looking good can burn off some calories during the spring and summer. Most household chores are treasure troves for staying in better shape.

Habit #52: Don't Shy Away from Post-Workout Snacks

Your body will be pretty drained after an intense workout. Eating a small amount of food will help to regain some of those crucial nutrients lost when working out while keeping your metabolism up and you feeling great.

Picking your snack can make a huge difference, too. Something rich in protein (like beans or nuts) will build muscle for your body, while something a bit leaner (like fruits) will give your body a bit of sugar it might have lost.

Above all snacks, you should always drink water before, during, and after your workouts. The worst thing you can do to stay healthy is let yourself become dehydrated. Keep a water bottle filled throughout the day and make sure to drink at least a gallon every 24 hours.

Chapter 3: Healthy Eating Habits

While working out and exercising is great to stay fit and keep your weight down, your eating habits dictate how much weight you gain or lose over long periods of time. Similar to your exercising habits, healthy eating habits won't affect you or your healthy immediately. Rather, they will take time to show any lasting results. That said, like all habits, these take time to develop as a part of your normal routine.

Eating habits are similar to exercising habits in many ways, but they must be approached differently because how you interact with food and eating said food is inherently different than how you interact with exercise on a day to day basis.

Habit #53: Know How to Change Your Habits Safely

Dieting, or even minor changes to your eating habits on a daily basis have the chance to be problematic in the long run if you don't know what you're doing. That's why it's essentially you consider your lifestyle before changing your habits.

Eating too little (especially while adjusting your exercise routine) can cause you to suffer from a lack of daily calorie intake, while eating too much or not enough variety can lead to health issues later on.

Habit #54: Know Your Eating Goals

It's good to get into the habit of knowing your long-term goals before you start changing the way you live. If, for example, you begin to start eating less for the sake of losing weight, it's important to understand what then to eat so you don't miss a lot of essential nutrients in food (to avoid becoming malnourished).

Habit #55: Keep a Log of Foods You've Eaten

A big mistake people often make is not keeping track of what they put in their bodies. It's easy to say "I'll have just one burger" when you aren't sure the last time you had one. Keeping track of your daily intake of food allows you to monitor how healthy or unhealthy your food choices are over time as well as keeping track of variety, or a lack thereof, in your meal choices.

Like exercising, there are tons of apps and services out there that will keep track of your daily food intake for you… kind of. If you're willing to put in the food you eat day to day (and where you got the food if it's fast food), then many apps and services will fill in the rest for you.

Habit #56: Plan Meals in Advance

It's easy to make an excuse for fast food when you don't have dinner planned at home. If you begin each week planning the meals you want to eat each day or, if you want to go above and beyond, preparing some of said meals, you'll have less of an excuse to swing by McDonald's on the way home.

Planning meals in advance also allows you to note what foods you eat, or plan on eating, regularly so you can make changes before you even begin buying the ingredients.

Finding fun and tasty recipes (that are also easy) can be tricky. Sure, there's the internet and cookbooks, which are both great sources, those can take time and, like picking out a movie on Netflix, offer too many options to choose from.

In the back of this book, for your pleasure and ease of access, we've provided you five easy to try recipes that taste delicious. Whether you're making a meal for yourself, or for a group of friends, each recipe is worth trying out once (even if it's just to hone your skills in the kitchen).

Habit #57: Make a List and Stick to It

When you're ready to stock up on your food for the following week, it's important to plan out every ingredient you'll need.

Making a shopping list is an easy way to have all the ingredients in one place (whether it be on a post-it note or on your cell phone). It also prevents you from picking up any unnecessary sweets while preparing your healthier meals.

Making a list goes perfectly with planning your meals. If you only give yourself time to visit the grocery store once a week, you better go in with a week of meals planned and a strict list of what you need for each meal. Each trip to the grocery store is filled with temptation (sweets, ice cream, extra pasta, easy frozen meals, etc.). Don't let these unnecessary foods get to you. Go to the grocery store when you need to and stick to that list of yours.

Habit #58: Change it Up

Eat a variety of foods to keep your body balanced and healthy. While many people enjoy meat enough to have it at every meal, make sure to mix in fruits and vegetables to add balance and variety to each and every meal.

That doesn't mean you can't eat the same kind of food for every meal. Say you like tacos but don't want to eat the same old tacos day after day. Mix it up with turkey tacos the next day, or vegan tacos the next. Have fun with your variation of food and spend time to experiment with the foods you're familiar with.

Habit #59: Know Suitable Substitutions

Because variety is so important to keeping meals balanced and healthy, it's important to know other sources for key nutrients outside of the norm. For example, rather than relying on red meat to give you that boost of protein, look to beans for a different approach to receive the same nutrients. Beans, in this case, offer fiber as an additional bonus to the protein you would be receiving from meat.

Habit #60: Know the Benefits of Food Groups

I'm sure most people are familiar with the Food Pyramid, or what is now called the "MyPlate." Keeping the five basic food types in mind (Fruits, vegetables, grains, proteins, and dairy -- as well as fats and oils), you should learn what each food type has to offer in general nutrients and health benefits. Of course, not all fruits offer exactly the same thing, but each food group has general rules to guide your eating habits.

Habit #61: Know How Much Time You Have

Stay conscious of how much time you have to prepare and eat your meal. If you don't have a lot of time, make something small to tide you over. If you have a few hours to spare, consider spending that time to prepare a more balanced and full meal.

Planning your meal preparation time and time to eat around how much time you have will save you lots of stress and headaches. Allowing yourself time to eat will also help relieve that stress and give you that time to really consider your options.

Habit #62: Don't Over-Buy

Plan your meals so that you don't have a lot of extra food. If you want pasta for dinner one night, buy enough to feed yourself and whoever else is eating dinner with you. If you buy too much, you'll end up eating the same thing for several days in a row and that's a quick way to get sick of your favorite foods.

Habit #63: Don't Shop Hungry

Plan your trips to the store around your meals. Go shopping after you've eaten so you can think about what you need without your hunger getting in your way.

In an earlier habit, we mention the temptations at the grocery store. These temptations will only intensify if you go through those glass doors with a rumbling stomach. Oddly similar to working out, eat an hour or so before shopping to allow your body to fully digest your food (but soon enough after to not be hungry again). This will save you money and from regret from buying food you don't need to later on.

Habit #64: Eat Smaller Meals, More Frequently

Big meals are common, especially around the holiday season. Don't be fooled by their appeal though. You want to eat smaller meals throughout the day, not three large ones. It's a common suggestion for people to eat five meals throughout the day that are about half the size of a normal meal. This way your metabolism stays constantly high all day without that inevitable food coma.

Habit #65: Note Your Portion Sizes

A portion of food is often a lot smaller than you think. Especially here in the USA where food comes big. Note what a portion size should be and base your intake on that.

Noting your portion size can also go hand in hand with monitoring the food you're eating. If you're eating pasta, a serving of plain noodles will be larger than a serving of noodles with meat sauce. Consider your meals as a whole to really figure out serving size. Don't eat a full serving of steak and a full serving of chicken and consider it balanced.

Habit #66: Balance Your Eating Habits with Your Exercise Habits

Both Eating healthy and exercising are required to keep a healthy lifestyle. If you exercise more than the average person, you burn more calories, and can therefore eat more. The same can be said about the other way around. If you don't exercise as much as you think your should, don't eat a lot either.

Habit #67: Buy Fresh

When given an option, buy fresh over frozen or pre-packaged,

This applies especially to Meat. While some foods can stand being frozen and not lose a lot of their nutrients (like fruits and vegetables), fresh is always a better option for taste.

There are times when fresh foods are not available (depending on the season, your region, and if there's a lack or surplus of whatever food you're looking for). There are tons of variables that determine if you can find fresh food where you live. Keep an eye out for fresh foods at your local grocery store or, better yet, your local farmer's market for the best deals.

Habit #68: Avoid Preserved Food

Preservatives are the enemy when looking for healthy foods, especially with fried foods. Preservatives, eaten too much, can lead to cancer.

*Yes, preservatives can lead to colon cancer, but it requires a lot of preservatives and bad luck. I'm not saying you will definitely get cancer if you eat one frozen chicken wing, but eating them enough will increase your chances.

Habit #69: Eat Breakfast

Breakfast is the start of your day, it only makes sense you fuel up. Eating breakfast will give you the energy you need and help you wake up.

Habit #70: Check The Labels

Check out the labels on the foods your buy. Keeping track of what ingredients are in each food and what and how much of each nutrient are in it.

Habit #71: Tune your Tastebuds

Many foods many people enjoy (coffee, tea, chocolate) usually come sweetened with sugar or other artificial sweeteners. You can train your taste buds to not want all that sugar in your drinks and sweets.

Instead of milk chocolate, buy dark cocoa. Instead of a Starbuck's Vanilla Latte Frappuccino, drink black coffee. Chances are, your taste buds aren't huge fans of the bitterness right away, but you can train them to like it over super sweet foods and drinks.

Habit #72: Eat Slower

Physically eating your food slower will give your body time to let your brain know that it's full. It takes about ten minutes for your body and mind to begin to signal to you that you're ready to stop eating.

Eating slow means more time to enjoy your food and more time for your body to signal that it's ready to stop.

Habit #73: Cut Out Super Sweet Beverages

As hard as it is, remove all soda from your diet. Soda is nothing but sugar and water and more sugar. It does nothing to benefit you and is designed to be addictive.

Habit #74: Find Healthy Foods to Satisfy Your Sweet Tooth

When you do cut out deep fried foods, snacks, and soda, find something to replace them to satisfy your needs. Baked chips, dark chocolate, nuts and grains, and water flavors are great ways to satisfy your sweet tooth needs.

Habit #75: Slow Down and Consider Your Options

When planning meals, or when driving home to begin preparing food, consider your options for your meals. It's too easy to pick up unhealthy-but-easy food when you don't weigh your options.

Chapter 4: General Health Habits

Exercise and healthy eating are essential to keeping a healthy lifestyle, but there are many other habits you can do to help aid you in both. These range from simple habits like setting reminders, to habits that require more thought such as practicing better posture.

These following habits are designed to help you live healthier, but won't necessarily make you lose weight or feel healthier overall.

Habit #76: Keep a Calendar

Google Calendar and Apple Calendar are both great apps for keeping track of appointments, meals, events, birthday, and countless other things you many need to keep track of. Keeping a calendar helps you stay organized (both on paper and mentally) and will make it easy to double check your schedule when making new plans.

If a calendar on your phone or computer doesn't sound too appealing, use a paper one on your wall. It's your schedule, you get to decide how to organize it.

Habit #77: Spend Time Aware of Your Posture

Three to five times a day, consider how you're sitting at that moment. Chances are, your posture is not as good as it could be and it can be improved. When you consider it, adjust so that your back is straight and your feet are planted firmly on the ground. You're posture will remain this way for at least a few minutes.

Naturally, you'll find yourself considering it throughout the day and adjusting it accordingly. Eventually, you'll fix your posture without thinking about it making it a lifelong habit.

Habit #78: Meditate

Meditation can be used for several reasons, but most frequently is used to clear one's head or calm one down. Use a few minutes each day to spend time with your thoughts and forget about the world outside. The time alone will help you stay calm throughout the day.

Habit #79: Congratulate Yourself

As you complete your goals and do well in your everyday life, congratulate yourself. You earn a pat on the back and who better to give it to you than you yourself?

Habit #80: Treat Yourself First

There will be times that you need to put yourself first to stay stable. If you need a personal day to stay sane, take one. It's always good to put others' emotions first, but there will be times that that can't be the case for your own health.

Habit #81: Get Enough Sleep

Sleep helps your mind recharge. You'll notice a huge difference in your day if you make sure to get enough sleep each night. The amount of sleep you need is based off your age, sex, and other variables that your doctor can tell you about.

Habit #82: Don't Get Too Much Sleep

On the opposite side of the spectrum, getting too much sleep is almost as bad for you. If you sleep too much, too often, your body will adjust and assume it needs that much sleep to function. When that happens, you'll need that amount of sleep, meaning getting the proper amount of sleep will be too little for your body.

Habit #83: Go Outside

If you're not going outside to exercise, go out to get a breath of fresh air and some sun. Sun helps with your daily vitamins as well as reduces depression.

Habit #84: Talk to People

Humans are social creatures. That's a cliche, but it's also very true. Every day, make it a point to talk to someone, anyone, to get your fill. Even if you just say hello to your neighbor or mail-carrier, it can turn a day around instantly.

Habit #85: Spend Time With Yourself

Learn to be happy spending time with yourself. If you don't like hanging out by yourself, others will pick up on it.

Habit #86: Step Out of Your Comfort Zone

A little bit of stress can increase your heart rate and raise your adrenaline levels to get you pumped up. Use that increased adrenaline to your advantage.

Habit #87: Work First, Play Later

Get any work done first so you can play later. If you finish your work early on, it won't become the center of your mind while you avoid it.

Fulfilling your responsibilities before having fun will allow you less stress and more time to enjoy yourself.

Habit #88: Reflect

Every day, find times to reflect on your day. Consider what you did well and what you can improve on, your mistakes and victories, if you overcame a challenge or if you couldn't figure out a problem. Spend time considering what you did well and what you can do in the future to better how you handled a situation.

Habit #89: Be Flexible

Life never goes according to plan. You can plan out weeks in advance and, chances are, something will mess up those plans. Remains flexible and willing to alter your schedule to make life easier on yourself. If you prepare yourself mentally for changes that may occur, when plans do go awry, you won't be as stressed.

Habit #90: Be Emotional Sometimes

This one is frowned upon, especially for all you men out there. Emotions are usually seen as weird or off putting, especially in public. The truth is, we all have emotions and keeping them locked up will only cause them to build and lead to unhealthy outlets. Let out emotions when you need to. Watch a sad movie every once and awhile and cry. There's no shame.

Habit #91: Laugh

Whether something legitimately makes you laugh or not, find a reason to. Laughter releases endorphins in your brain, which make you happier. If you can't find anything to laugh about, fake it. Fake laughter has the potential to real laughter.

Habit #92: Make Mistakes

One of the biggest problems with school systems today is an emphasis on knowing the correct answers. You're going to make mistakes in life no matter what you do. Allow yourself mistakes every now and again and learn from them.

Habit #93: Have a Hobby at All Times

Having a hobby not only gives you something to do when you're bored, it also allows you a trait to tie to your identity. You may not be "the guy with the poodle" or "the girl who can dance," but you'll always have something that you can practice and get better at.

Habit #94: Don't Compare Yourself to You

Too many times, people have distorted views of themselves.

Understand that every flaw you see in yourself, every minor little error in your face, is most likely invisible to those around you.

Everyone has flaws they don't like about themselves, and focusing on them will drive you to depression.

Habit #95: Be Nice to People

This one may seem pretty obvious, but it's something people forget to do more often than not. Being nice to other people for the sake of being nice makes you feel better as well. Sure, this can be seen as a selfish reason to be nice, but if making someone else feel better, it's ok to feel good about it.

Remember, even a small little compliment to someone you've never talked to has the potential to put them in a happy mood for the rest of the day.

Chapter 5: Healthy Recipes

Some of the easiest habits come in the form of knowing what to cook when you want a healthy meal. Included in the next section are five recipes to get you started planning, preparing, and cooking up fresh foods to help you, your friends, and your family eat healthier and feel better. The recipes provided are fan-favorites from a variety of regions and countries, and use several different cooking methods.

Recipe #1: One-Pan Vegetables with Sausage

If you're not a fan of vegetables but need to find a way to fit them into your diet, try mixing them in with some tasty meat to help mix or even mask the flavors.

This recipe offers a great variety of food groups (with their own unique nutrients to offer) to help your meal stay balanced with little effort. While this specific recipe offers ease of balance and health, it offers one other aspect that makes it especially easy: One pot.

Not only is it easy to cook, clean up is a breeze because, as the title suggests, all the food is prepared in one pot.

Preparation time: 10 minutes

Cooking time: 30 minutes

Necessary Ingredients:

Red Potato (2 cups)

Green beans (3/4 of a pound)

Broccoli (1 1/2 cups)

2 Large Bell Peppers

Sausage (10 ounces)

Olive oil (6 Tablespoons)

Red pepper flakes (only if you want a bit of spice)

Paprika (1 teaspoon)

Garlic powder (1/2 Tablespoon)

Oregano (1 Tablespoon)

Parsley (1 Tablespoon)

Salt (a pinch)

Pepper to taste

Directions:

Preheat your oven to 400 degrees fahrenheit.

Place Foil over a baking sheet.

Cut the potatoes into small pieces (the smaller and more consistent the pieces are in size, the quicker and more evenly they will cook). Trim the green beans and cut in half down the middle. Cut the broccoli and peppers. Finally, cut the sausage into small discs.

Place all of your cut ingredients onto your baking sheet. Sprinkle your spices on top and pour the olive oil over it. Mix your food on the baking sheet and make sure the olive oil and spices cover every last piece.

Bake your mixture for 15 minutes. Take your food from the oven and mix to make sure everything cooks evenly, then return it to the oven for 10 - 15 more minutes. Remove and enjoy!

Recipe #2: Vegan Jambalaya

Preparation time: 20 minutes

Cook time: 45 minutes

Vegan food often times gets a bad rap. People assume that just because something is vegan, it doesn't offer you all the necessary nutrients to be well-balanced or healthy. While it's true that most non-meat foods don't have a healthy amount of protein, there are several that help you get everything you need.

If you don't think the below recipe offers you enough protein, or simply won't fill you up, try adding beans or tofu. Both will add a bit more "meat" so to speak to your food to help fill you up faster. Without either, the recipe is delicious regardless and will surely change the way you view vegan food from here on out.

Necessary Ingredients:

Olive oil (3 Tablespoons)

Yellow onion (1 large)

Garlic (3 cloves)

Celery (4 stalks)

Tomatoes (4 cups)

Brown rice, uncooked (2 cups)

Vegetable stock (5 cups)

Bay leaves (3 leaves)

Paprika (1 teaspoon)

Hot sauce (2 teaspoons)

Salt (1 pinch)

Pepper (1 pinch)

Cilantro (3 Tablespoons)

Directions:

In a large skillet, heat the olive oil over medium heat.

Cut your onion, garlic, celery, and place into the heated oil. Sauté the vegetables for 3 - 4 minutes.

Slice your tomatoes and add them to your vegetables. Stir and let the mixture sit for one minute until soft.

Pour in your brown rice, vegetable stock, bay leaves, paprika, hot sauce, salt, and pepper to the mixture and stir to combine.

Cover with a tight lid and bring to a simmer.

Let your mixture simmer for 20-40 minutes.

Stir in fresh cilantro and serve.

Recipe #3: Tuscan White Bean Skillet

A big part of eating healthier is being creative with the food you prepare. Bringing in inspiration from other countries of the world is a great way to try new things while staying reasonably healthy.

Italy has always had a wide variety of flavors to add to your palate (flavors outside of Olive Garden). While the food can take longer to make, usually, this White Bean Salad is delicious, good for you, and only takes about half an hour, making it a great combination for anyone trying to add new meals to their weeknight tables.

Ingredients:

Olive oil (2 Tablespoons)

Brown mushrooms (8 ounces)

Yellow onion (1 large onion)

Garlic (3 cloves)

Sun dried tomatoes (2/3 cup)

Fire-roasted diced tomatoes (2 cans)

Cannellini beans (2 cans)

Quartered artichoke hearts (1 can)

Kosher salt (1/2 teaspoon)

Black pepper (1/2 teaspoon)

Oregano (1 teaspoon)

Thyme (1/2 teaspoon)

Sugar (1 teaspoon)

Directions:

In a skillet, heat 1 tablespoon over medium-high heat (about 7 for those of you with a 1 - 10 knob). Wait for the oil to simmer.

Cut your mushrooms into slices and place one layer in the oil. Cook each side of the mushroom slices for about a minute and a half, then remove and add to a large bowl. Do this until all your mushrooms are browned.

Add the other tablespoon of olive oil to your skillet and add the onions. Keep moving for about 3 minutes.

Add the sun-dried tomatoes and chopped garlic to the skillet. Cook until The smell fills your kitchen (about 2 minutes).

Add the diced tomatoes, beans, artichoke hearts, salt, pepper, oregano, thyme, and sugar. Stir until combined and cover the pan.

Cook for ten minutes and serve.

Recipe #4: Chicken Tacos

So many people in the USA love going out to grab a bite to eat. Chipotle, Taco Bell, Del Taco, etc. are all examples of Mexican (or, at least, Mexican-American) cuisine. While you could argue that these restaurants offer tasty food for a reasonable price, they are not the most healthy options for you. In fact, many of the food is some of the worst options for you.

That doesn't mean you need to cut all Mexican-inspired food from your diet. It means that exact opposite, actually. This is your chance to find recipes that satisfy your south-of-the-border needs, but don't add inches to your waist.

The best part about the recipe below is its ease of cooking. If time is the most valuable part of the day, you're in luck! The chicken tacos use a slow cooker (or Crock Pot as many people know it) to cook your food over time, with little effort on your end. Leave it in the pot for a few hours while you clean, exercise, or even leave the house to run errands.

Necessary Ingredients:

Chicken breasts, skinless and boneless (2 pounds)

Taco seasoning mix (1 packet or equivalent)

Salsa (1 Jar)

Cilantro (1/3 cup)

Lime Juice (2 limes worth)

Directions:

First, place your full chicken breasts in the very bottom of your slow cooker. Sprinkle the tops of the breasts with your taco seasoning, salsa, lime juice, and cilantro.

Place (and if your slow cooker allows it, lock) the lid on the crock pot. Set the heat on high and cook for four hours (or set it to low and cook for 7 hours).

Once it's cooked, place the chicken breasts on a plate or cutting board and separate with two forks. Place the chicken in a bowl and pour about 1/2 cup of the leftover juice over the now-shredded chicken.

Serve with soft or hard shell taco shells and add toppings as you see fit. (Note: toppings have the amazing ability to add a lot of extra calories to your meals.)

Recipe #5: Breakfast Casserole

Advertising for the slow cooker is easy when they make meals so, well, easy. This next recipe is for those of you who hate waking up early to make a healthy breakfast. This recipe was designed specifically to allow you to let a nice, hearty breakfast cook overnight to be warm and ready for you as soon as you wake up. What's a better way to start a long day than eating a fresh, hot meal that you didn't even have to cook that morning?

Necessary Ingredients:

frozen shredded hash brown (30 ounces)

Ground sausage, cooked until brown (1/2 pound)

Bacon, cooked then chopped into small pieces (1 pound)

Cheddar cheese, shredded (2 cups)

Mozzarella cheese, shredded (1 cup)

1 onion

1 green pepper

1 red pepper

12 eggs

Milk (1/2 cup)

Salt (1 pinch)

Ground black pepper (1 pinch)

Sugar (1/8 teaspoon)

Directions:

Rub butter over the inside of your slow cooker.

Place half of your frozen hash browns into the bottom of the pot and top with your cooked sausage, cooked bacon pieces, shredded cheese, sliced onions, chopped green and red peppers.

Place another layer of hash browns on top of your ingredients.

Whisk your dozen eggs and mix in sugar and milk. Add salt and pepper and mix everything one last time.

Pour your egg mixture over your layered hash browns in the crock pot and cook on low for 8 hours.

If you want to try this recipe, but don't want to wait over night, you can also set the heat to high and let it cook for 4 hours.

Thank You

Thank you for picking up "100 Easy but Powerful Diet Habits: Powerful, Healthy Habits that lead to major weight loss and change your life" from your digital library or store. WE sincerely hope that these habits become a part of your everyday life to help you become the healthier person you wish to be.

We'd like to thanks all of our chef friends for creating the recipes in this book and hope that they continue to be creative and posting on their respective blogs, websites, or video channels. All recipes belong to the creators and they deserve all credit for creating them.

Thank you again for picking up this book, and enjoy your new, easier, healthier lifestyle!

www.ingramcontent.com/pod-product-compliance
Lightning Source LLC
Chambersburg PA
CBHW060156290526
45789CB00003B/1059
* 9 7 8 1 5 4 2 3 7 2 8 2 4 *